# Yoga
# for Beginners

*Basic and strength poses. Weight loss, love your body. Best practical tips.*

INNA VOLIA

# Table of Contents

# Introduction

When the word yoga is mentioned, a lot of things come to mind however taking time to study the subject and understanding what it actually is can be quite liberating. Yoga is a science that I would highly recommend for virtually everyone who seems to be under the pressure of life to realize their goals faster while still remaining sober and focused. Yoga is a technique that has been proven to provide effective tools that not only enhance levels of flexibility, strength and self awareness, it also provides a sense of calm and fulfillment that cannot be achieved through conventional exercise methods.

It's a practice that cuts across many cultures and religions world over and has diverse benefits that are incomparable to any other form of exercising as it focuses on the whole person with all the spiritual, physical, emotional and mental aspects of the being well impacted by the practice. Yoga for Beginners is a book that' shared in detail all that yoga practice entails. Various aspects of yoga practice has been shared in detail with the topics like fundamentals of practicing yoga, benefits of yoga, meditation and the various yoga exercises being addressed in detail.

Take your time and read through the book so that you are well informed about the subject. The yoga and meditation exercises have been made simpler and much easier to understand, a fact that makes the book not to be only ideal for the beginners but those that have some basic knowledge can equally benefit from reading the book. I would advice that you read the book all through before coming back and practicing on the various exercises that are shared in the book. That's when you will have clarity on the results to expect and how you can schedule you exercises for great success.

Thank you for taking your time to download the book and enjoy your reading!

# Chapter 1

## Understanding Yoga

Yoga can be defined as a spiritual science that's aimed at self realization and entail use of the mind to control activities. Yoga can also be defined as a type of exercise in which you move your body into various positions in order to be more fit and flexible, so as to improve your breathing and to relax your mind. Yoga is considered as a practical aid and not religion. It's an ancient art which basically involve harmonizing development of the mind, spirit and the body. When one takes on to yoga fully one will be able to get a sense of peace and well being especially being in uniformity with the surrounding.

The methods of yoga encompass the entire fields of one's existence and that range from the emotional, physical, mental and spiritual. The physical bit of yoga is referred to as Hatha Yoga, which uses poses and predetermined breathing sequence which calls for concentration and discipline. Yoga can be practiced by all, irrespective of body size, age, and other physical abilities.  As much as it may be, there are certain complex postures that some do attain but that does not mean that it's restricted to such people but it is meant for everyone. Given that yoga involves physical exercise, it makes your body strong and also helps in improving the functioning of digestive, respiratory and some hormonal systems.

Yoga is essentially a spiritual subtle science discipline which is practiced with the intention of bringing harmony and to the body and mind.  It also enhances emotional strength and clarity of mind. The biggest thing about yoga is about self realization and self development. Yoga places you on a proactive path in your life and each time you tend to be on top

5

of situations around you and hence eliminating the reactive phase of life. For example, our daily lives can be filled with situations that cause worry and anxiety but by practicing yoga; one is able to gain clear focus regarding issues that may seem to be difficult and overwhelming.

With yoga one is able to visit some depth of spiritual matters that then hence reveals certain facets of life that one is not able to tune into on a normal life frequency. For example, gaining clear insight on how to handle an issue or the best steps to take can be made much easier by practicing yoga. As you practice yoga, you get to deal with very nitty gritty issues that usually get people unawares and most of the time becomes an impediment to progress. On the physical arena it enables you to become a mechanic so to say, to your body. You will end up reducing so much expense on medication because the body is already well tuned and toned too.

There is a lot that one can achieve with flexible body and muscles. Apart from being in great body weight, you also get to eliminate some of the diseases that can be associated with lack of physical health and well being. Attaining self realization through yoga therefore means that you're able to overcome all manner of suffering which then leads into a state of liberation for the mind, body and soul. As is always said prevention is better than cure which means that as you go about doing yoga apart from the spiritual angle of it, you will end up with a much more healthy body which will be easier to treat because the ailments you may experience are bordering on injury and not lifestyle diseases. Yoga generally brings balance to the body systems and to wider aspect also makes one to be alert with the foods that we eat.

# History of Yoga

Many historians tend to put it that yoga is dating back about 5000 years ago. They do suggest that yoga must have emanated from the Stone Age era of Shamanism in the orient nations. This is in countries of India, Afghanistan and Pakistan because most of Hindu religious symbols, rituals and ideas seem to have originated from this part of the world before they spread to other lands. The ancient intention of yoga was for the purpose of trying to understand the cosmic order through inward experience. These people wanted to experience certain understanding of the cosmos for their good.

The word yoga was derived from the root Yuj, meaning to join, unite or yoke. According to the yogic scriptures, practicing yoga is believed lead to the union of one's consciousness with the universal consciousness.  Such a union expressed a perfect harmony for the body and mind. Modern scientists have expressed that all things within the universe manifests a similar quantum firmament and a person who gets to experience this level of oneness is said to be in yoga.  This is now what later turned yoga into a much more spiritual thing than what it was before, and from there it was considered more as a way of individual enlightenment and salvation.

The practice of yoga is said to have started at the dawn of civilization with its origin stretching to thousands of years ago before the onset of religion or belief system. It's said that between the period 500 BC – 800 AD, the practice of yoga became quite prominent in regards to the history and development of yoga. However its origin can be traced to the banks of Lake Kantisarovar in Himalayas where the founder Adiyogi shared his knowledge with seven sages. The sages then carried the yogic science to various parts of the world which included Asia, South America, Middle East and Northern

Africa. It was however in India where the Yogic science realized its fullest expression.

The presence of yoga has infiltrated Indian folk traditions, Vedic and Upanishadic, Civilization and the Indian heritage. Yoga has been expressed through various mystical expressions of the South Asian tradition. Today yoga has permeated several cultures and languages such as Hindi, Tibet, Tamil, Sanskrit, Prakit and Marathi amongst others. It's also penetrated religions like Hinduism, Buddhists, Jainism, and even the western cultures. Yoga is currently viewed as the most widespread spiritual practice in the world with the ultimate focus being peace.

# Practicing Yoga

Once you understand what yoga is all about, there is always a strong desire to get into the practice however there are factors that should be put into consideration before starting off. Yoga classes and lessons are rapidly spreading and this can be found in various places across cities like in gyms, karate training halls and other public halls where youth usually meet for extra curriculum activities. At some point it's fused with salsa dance lessons just to make it more appealing and impactful.

There are numerous factors that should be put into consideration before starting off with practicing yoga; below are some of them.

## 1. The yoga teacher

One thing that should influence the place where you take your yoga practice is the yoga teacher. There are different types of teachers and how they are aligned with some being of high energy, alignment focused, spiritual based or calming. It's important that you understand what your priority is and the results you intend to get as that should guide you to the teacher that best suits you.

## 2. The class atmosphere

Another factor that you should consider is the class atmosphere as it can greatly affect your yoga practice. Being in a class with people that are open-minded provides a great atmosphere for learning and growing. Most people also prefer a class atmosphere where the community practices conscious living.

### 3. The class style

When it comes to practicing yoga, there are various styles that one can incorporate. Taking up yoga practices in a class that engages in faster paced practice can be of great help.

### 4. Cost

Another factor that's worth considering is the cost of the yoga practice. Affordability is a key factor as engaging into something that you may not sustain in the long run can negatively impact your training process. The amount charged for the yoga lessons per month or per session vary depending on the teacher and other factors. It's better to consider choosing monetary value that you get from the practice instead of going for lavish membership.

### 5. A meditation aspect

The fact that majority of the yoga classes incorporate meditation also contributes to it as a factor that should be considered. As you learn yoga, you also get to enhance your meditation skills which is quite vital given meditation is something that's practiced by many.

### 6. Convenience

This is another factor that should be considered considering the fact that you need to engage in the practice several days within the week. You will need a place that's easy to access in regards to location and the length of time that you may take to access the place.

There are various health benefits that are associated with engaging in yoga practice and even as one enrolls for the practice, they should be clear on the benefits to expect. Yoga practice has been embraced world over and is continually being embraced by many celebrities in the west as an appropriate wellness exercise. So far yoga has broken the stereotype that getting involved into it is a form of worshipping the gods of the east. The practice so far cuts across all divides, class and lifestyles and some basic knowledge about the practice is important for maximum benefits.

The other thing with yoga is that it involves a lot of precision, that calls for awareness involved and on a wider perspective the growth and success that is registered in physical, mental and emotional areas of a person. The perfection needed will be dependent on practice, having determination coupled with a lot of effort. In summary yoga will get you into great shape, hence making you feel and look younger and full of energy with a constantly clear mind and focus. It's capable of bringing you to a place of achieving better results through meditation as you get to practice being calm and united in spirit with the universe.

Americans define yoga as a mystic and Hindu discipline which one undertakes to achieve self liberation and getting in unity with the supreme spirit or universe. It ensures deliberate and intensive concentration and deep meditation while at certain postures coupled with predetermined breathing. Apart from the societies that yoga practice has existed for so long to the extent that it may be regarded as a normal thing to do, those who are new to yoga should ensure that they get clear understanding regarding the practice even as they engage in some training if success with the practice is to be realized.

# Chapter 2

## The Fundamentals of Practicing Yoga

Yoga works according to one's emotional, energy, mind and body level and this has led to yoga being classified into four categories. Karma yoga entails use of body, bhakti yoga involves use of emotions, gyana yoga entails use of the mind and the intellect and kriya yoga which entails use of energy. Each system of yoga that people get to practice falls in the four categories of yoga and can either involve one or more of the categories. When planning of practicing yoga, it's vital that you work with a guru as only a guru can be able to mix the ideal combination for the four fundamental paths which is important for effective yoga practice.

Yoga education and practice has been passed down by experienced and knowledgeable gurus and the education is focused towards taking care of an individual's entire being. It's presumed that a good, highly balanced and well integrated individual is more useful to not only the individual but entire family and society at large. There are numerous yoga institutions worldwide where yoga education and practice is undertaken and millions of people across the world have benefitted from yoga practice. Yoga practice is considered as an orientation to healthy living and worth practicing by all regardless of one's religion, race or nationality.

# Stages of Yoga

There are several benefits that can be attributed to yoga with the primary one being moksha (liberation). At some point, the benefits of yoga may be directly derived from its principle meanings. Yoga as a disciplined way to attaining a goal, it brings the discipline much needed for achieving goals. At the same time getting to master the techniques that will help you to control your body and mind most of the time. When one can perfect the art of helping our minds to focus on a particular thing, then the sharper the focus the easier it is to be able to realize success in that particular area.

From time to time over the ages the purposes or principles of yoga have experienced variations in various ways. So far yoga should be a meditative means of redeeming dysfunctional perception and cognition at the same time being able to come to a point whereby you overcome and release yourself from any form of suffering thereby realizing inner peace and salvation or rather deliverance. Yoga is also viewed as a path of the supernatural whereby you get to come to the knowledge of some realities that cannot be accessed in the ordinary. It's also viewed as a technique of acquiring the capacity to gain entry into other bodies by being able to generate multiple bodies and being able to attain some other supernatural states.

Yoga is also seen as a technique of being able to raise and expand the consciousness and be able to extend to the point of being with everything and all things. There are various ailments that are being said that can be brought under control by engaging in yoga. Now each type of ailment or condition will need a unique yoga style. Therefore it's necessary to understand the various types of yoga so as to engage with adequate knowledge.

## Types of Yoga

There are various types of yoga and each one has got a way of how it functions which then identifies with a particular approach to life. One type of yoga may be much more convenient to one person than another. But the most important thing with yoga is that all of these paths have a way by which it is able to overlap hence no need to think that may be what you are dealing with is not the best.

## Raja yoga

The term raja means royal and this type of yoga mainly centers on meditation. This involves very stern adherence to the so called eight limbs or stages of yoga. These stages take the following order; ethical standards, yama; self-discipline, niyama; posture which is asana; extension of breadth or control of breadth, pranayama; sensory withdrawal, pratyahara; concentration, dharana; meditation, dhyana and ecstatic point which is Samadhi. This yoga usually befits those who love searching inwards hence meditation. This type of yoga is common with religious members and spiritual communities who can be associated with the royal class.

## Karma yoga

This is also being called the path of service. The ideology here is collected from the school of thought that our life experience today is like a sum total of our past actions. Therefore the actions we get engaged in today determine what we are going to experience in the future. Basically karma is more inclined to the branch of public service to humanity, which is a selfless service and in line with volunteer situations.

## Bhakti Yoga

This is a path of devotion which mostly sees the divine in creation and always channels emotions positively. With bhakti yoga one is able to cultivate being accepted and be able develops tolerance for everyone they come around. In this yoga, the yogis (those who practice yoga) tend to develop a devotional nature of their path in all thought, speech and doings. People like Mahatma Gandhi are considered to have exhibited these qualities and the same alluded to Martin Luther King, Jr. Mother Teresa was a mix between karma and Bhakti which focuses on devotion and service.

## Jnana Yoga

This is considered to be yoga of the mind which is bordering on wisdom and it is the path for scholars or academicians. This yoga demands developing the intellect by study of materials and texts based on yogic tradition. It is the toughest but the most direct, its fit for those who are good at academics because of a lot of studies involved. This yoga cuts across all that are inclined to deep religion.

## Tantra Yoga

This yoga takes a ritualistic pathway which encompasses consecration of sexuality. This in a wider sense is a more ritualistic approach to almost all aspects of life. For those that get into it they are encouraged to stay celibate because much of this is around sexual ritual. It is said that this group of people are prone to obtaining extra ordinary results in all that they do, be it some Japanese tea ceremony, or even the consecration of sacrament in a catholic preaching service.

Tantra yoga is the most esoteric and appeals to those who enjoy feminine principles that are associated with the cosmos.

Many tantric yogis are known to find extreme fulfillment in ceremonies

## Ashtanga Yoga

Ashtanga is one of the most commonly practiced yoga today and it means eight. Ashtanga yoga is a step by step guide to achieving meaningful and purpose oriented life. It based on all around ethical conduct and self discipline; as much as the emphasis is in health it also covers spiritual aspects as well. The eight steps (limbs) acts as a guide towards living a meaningful and purposeful life. Each limb in this yoga has what it deals with and the first limb is yama

**Yama**: Yama focuses on ethical standards and integrity. It also boarder on behavior and overall conduct of a person. Yama is mindful of the feeling of others and helps with acknowledgement of some of the spiritual aspects of nature. It's based on the golden rule of "doing unto others what you would have them do unto you".

**Niyama**: This is the second limb and it focuses on self-discipline and spiritual focus. It is evident in situations like regular spiritual involvements like visiting houses of worship, consciously blessing your meals just before eating and on a regular basis getting some solitary time to wind off a day. This could be by taking a walk or sitting somewhere around a swimming pool or sitting somewhere in the balcony.

**Asanas:** Asanas is the third limb and it's more of some spiritual weeding whereby you engage in caring for the spirit which is embodied by the body. According to the yogic view, the body is seen as the temple of the spirit and taking care of it enhances spiritual growth. It is viewed that as the spirit grows, discipline is inculcated and concentration is enhanced thereby providing quality meditation. This stage comprises of techniques that are meant to enable one gain mastery over their respiratory process. This is achieved by recognizing the existing connection between the mind, breath and emotions.

**Pranayama yoga**: This is the fourth limb which deals with respiratory control or breathing sequence, because there is an interconnection between the mind, emotions and breath. This is a life force extension which can be practiced by doing power breathing exercises. This can be done all alone or incorporated with other forms of yoga preferably hatha yoga routine.

Up to that level you may realize that this yoga have majorly dealt with polishing our personalities, having control over the body, and strengthening of the mind while harnessing an individual's energy. Once these areas are done with then the next phase will basically involve how to perfect your best by accessing a higher state of existence.

**Pratyahara yoga:** The next step is called Pratyahara which is fifth limb or stage which means withdrawal or engaging in sensory transcendence. It involves a form of withdrawal and emancipation of one's mind from being dominated by sensual things and external things. The withdrawal aspect to objectively look out for habits that can be detrimental to one's health. It also provides a platform and an opportunity to take some position of rest and have a critical look at yourself. It also assists you in identifying your common craving, which may be a setback to your health and might in the long run interfere with inner growth.

Being in this state provides insulation of adoration by connecting your mind to that of the creator who made things of his desire. In actual sense the mind is usually the source and cause of bondage and same to liberation. It's bondage when the focus is on objects and its liberation when the focus is removed from the objects. Bondage sets in when the mind craves,

17

grieves and feels unhappy about something. Freedom comes when the mind is cleared of desires and fears. The argument in here is that both good and bad happens to human beings and therefore a choice has to be made on how to handle each situation.

When you want good then go for it but ensure that you have control not to crave for perfect because that will be a source of anxiety. This then means that the path or capacity to getting ruined or obtaining salvation is embedded within us.

According to the Hindu philosophy, being conscious is in three ways namely sattva, Rajas and Tamas.

- Sattva is the conscious state of being illuminated and pure or in good quality, which actualizes into clarity and mental serenity.

- Rajas is being in a state of mobility or being active which makes one to be active, and energetic and may be tensed and also willful.

- Tamas is the dark and restraining ability which in essence obstructs and counters the ability of rajas to work and sattva being able to reveal. Tamas is considered as a state of delusion and ignorance and when one is in this state, it's just in an inert state.

## Understanding three aspects of Consciousness

Therefore sattva is considered as the highway to divine while tamas is considered as demonic and rajas being the middle ground of the two. According to predominating guna, qualities or attributes will determine the faith one upholds, the food, sacrifices done and even the gifts one shares. Anyone born of divine is fearless, generous and with self control. Most of the time he will be truthful and free from anger, will show malice to nobody and show charity to all.

A person with attributes of Raja will tend to have inner thirst, passionate, will show level of covetousness and also hurt others in the process. They are filled with lust, and hatred, has envy and deceit. The desires are wild and insatiable, may be very easy to distract though ambitious and hungry to acquire things. This character will be uncomfortable with unpleasant things yet cling to good ones. The one with Tamas qualities will exhibit the demonic tendencies like he will be insolent, self conceited and full of deceit. Wrath, ignorance and run away cruelty are with him. Such like personalities do not know anything to do with purity and even right conduct much of their life is pleasure bordering on hell.

**Dharana:** This is purely concentration; it basically takes yogi deeper into his soul. At this point one doesn't look heaven ward to access God but rather looks inward. The very last 3 stages are geared to keep harmony with self and God. Through extended meditation, the knower, the knowledge and the known become one. The same applies to the seer, sight and the seen all lumps together. It's good for a man to get to differentiate the real from not real, the eternal from the transient and good from pleasant by discernment and wisdom.

Mind is considered king of the senses and one who has conquered his mind, senses and passion is considered king like

19

raja yoga, which is considered as a royal union with God who has inner light. Conquering the mind is king, and therefore a king should reach certain level of self master in the mind that ushers in the eight limb yoga. The eight limb yoga point is regarded as the complete mastery of self and may be considered as a science of kingly Yoga. Given that the central effect of yoga is through the mind, it's important to understand what to do to modify the mind. There are five classes or stages of modification of the mind and they are as follows:

i. **Pramana**: This is a standard or ideal situation which aids in measuring of the things or values by the mind. These may take the form of direct evidence like perception, deduction, or a word from an authority which can be found to be reliable and trustworthy.

ii. **Viparyaya**: This is a mistaken view which is observed only after some study to prove otherwise.

iii. **Vikalpa**: This is imagination which rests on verbal expression but do not have facts. For example a case whereby you are poor and very broke and you imagine operating a fat bank account with millions of Euros. The flip side of the thought is a rich chap thinking that he is poor.

iv. **Nidra:** Which is sleep and in this case there are no ideas or even experiences. This is the state we are in when we are asleep. You cannot recall your name, relatives many other things you are totally unconscious of. Therefore when one is able to get sound sleep then he wakes up refreshed.

v. **Smrti**: This is a situation of leaving in the past in that they are affected by the experiences of the past either positively or negatively. So by invoking those memories of the past they are hindered from the reality of a new day and possible new and better results.

There are also the aspect of trigger of pain which are as a result of the following:

- Ignorance or the doctrine that nothing is knowable.
- A strong individual feeling which isolates one from a group, this may be physical, intellectual, emotional or mental.
- Passion or attachment
- Repulsion or aversion
- Love and strong desire for life, though with a level of fear that one may be cut short from full enjoyment by death.

## Obstacles and Distractions

It is important that as one intends to get into yoga practice it's also important to know the forms of distractions and obstacles that may hinder you from the success of it.

1. A sickness that may affect the physical balance since it's the body that achieves the results that yoga brings. So any ill heath of the body will definitely hinder one from realizing the results of yoga as concentration is required while meditating.

2. Weakness of the body or mind that is so heavy that you may not feel comfortable to embrace any work. This blinds the goal, lack of clear path to follow.

3. Lack of clear decision and doubt. Yoga needs wisdom, faith, and assurance of the person engaging in the practice. When such is absent then the

achieving the ultimate goal becomes very difficult. As faith grows in the heart it should knock out lust, mental slowness, ill-intent and pride.

4. Laziness is another factor that can hinder one from realizing the benefits of yoga practice. The antidote to laziness is enthusiasm; hope should be kept alive and dispel hate and sorrow. And now with faith and enthusiasm, one is in a position to overcome resigned state of the body and mind.

5. False knowledge or illusion can also hinder one from benefiting from yoga practice. False knowledge will make one to feel that they are on the right path yet not, the way out for such a person is sitting in the right company of mature souls who can be able to guide the weak person to set foot strongly and get to the right path to overcome his weakness.

6. Falling short of ensuring continuity of a thought or the needed concentration which should then manifest into full reality. When you cannot overcome the problem of lack of concentration, then you cannot seek reality. When one is able to set eye on reality then clarity is guaranteed.

7. Just slipping off the concentration which has really taken you time to attain after a long practice. In yoga consistency is a major key to success of everything and when you have worked so hard it is not good to lose the sight of reality. This can occur when one decides to rejoice around smaller achievements and become lazy in doing practice hence short-circuiting the real deal. To revert back, it may call for waiting for divine grace to fall again because to access God you need to seek him and not relying on studies,

intellect but a stronger longing in your heart for him to manifest.

8. Insensibility and lack of enthusiasm can also distract one from realizing the benefits of practicing yoga. This is a case of self exaltation and self conceitedness. Such a person is always blind to the glory of God and also can hear from God. Usually they show very selfish traits and personal glory.

9. Being in a state whereby sensory stuff possesses the mind can also be a hindrance. In this case there is a strong longing for sensory things after they had been left behind and the feeling can be quite overwhelming. One can only get freedom by withdrawing and emancipation of the mind from domination of the senses and external things.

10. Other distractions are misery, despair, uncoordinated breathing and shaky body.

# Clearing the Misconceptions Associated with Practicing Yoga

There are numerous misconceptions that have been associated with practicing yoga and as a beginner, it's important that you understand them in order to avoid any confusion that might arise. When practicing yoga it's good to know that there are no absolutes as what may work for one person may not effectively work for another person. Yoga is a versatile practice and can be modified to suit any given need or taste. Below are some of the misconceptions that have been associated with practicing yoga.

## 1.  Yoga practice is for flexible people

As much as practicing some yoga postures may require a flexible body one of the first rules in yoga practice is to engage only in postures that your body, mind and spirit are comfortable with. So flexibility has nothing to do with practicing yoga. Good instructors understand that there may be variability in regards to flexibility of the participants and are able to guide accordingly through the practice process. It important to note that when it comes to practicing yoga, there are no rules, judgments or expectations.

## 2.  Yoga is a spiritual practice

Many people associate the practice of yoga to Eastern religion and some who would have wanted to practice it shy away due to that fact. It's however important to note that yoga does not adhere to a particular religion, community or belief system. It should be approached as an inner wellbeing technology. It's therefore possible to enjoy the benefits associated with practicing yoga even if you don't belong to any faith.

### 3. Yoga is too slow

When compared to other forms of exercises. Some people assume that yoga is quite slow and not effective for cardiovascular workout. This is not true as some of the yoga exercises can be quite intense. A practice like of power yoga is quite aerobic in nature and is known to induce strength. On the other hand executing postures effectively require coordination and flexibility alongside high levels of endurance which is not as slow as imagined.

### 4. Yoga is a competitive sport

There are some people who assume that yoga is a competitive sport and therefore shy away from the practice. As much as some of the important aspects of yoga consist of engagement in physical postures practice, it's actually a science that's aimed at enhancing, physical, spiritual and mental aspects of an individual. Yoga exercises may include some element of stretching that's familiar with some sport activities but that doesn't make it to become a competitive sport. The postures practiced in yoga are just a segment of what the entire program entails.

### 5. Yoga is for those who are fit

It's important to note that practicing yoga does not require any level of fitness to be attained before starting off with the exercise. Anybody can practice yoga regardless of their shape or sizes. If you are able to breathe then you can also do yoga and for effective engagement you should engage in exercises that complement your level of fitness. Regardless of your level of fitness you will be able to find class options that may be less vigorous and fits you well. To adjust to the intensity of the exercises without feeling hurt, you need to engage in more exercises before starting out on yoga practice so that you become more flexible in the process.

## 6. Yoga if for women

This is another misconception that can keep many from practicing yoga. As much as majority of those who practice yoga in some parts of the world tends to be women, it's a practice that can be embraced by both men and women. The benefit is great and is something that everyone can enjoy. Practicing yoga has a way of relaxing and rejuvenating the mind by giving it the ability to overcome negative feelings.

## 7. You must be in special yoga clothes

As much as being in yoga clothes is good, it should not be a hindrance to practicing yoga. You can enjoy practicing yoga even in any clothes as long as they are comfortable enough for the exercise.

# Chapter 3

## Benefits of Yoga

The main purpose of practicing yoga is to enable both the body and mind to develop awareness, strength and harmony. There are physical benefits as well as mental benefits that can be derived from practicing yoga. The physical poses and turns of the body are more of physical exercises which also keep the body fit. The relaxation techniques that are practiced helps with addressing various physical problems that the body could be experiencing. There are types of yoga that go deeper to address ailments like headaches, depression, menstrual irregularities amongst others.

Practicing yoga helps with changing the patterns of the nervous system which then causes the body fluids and the blood gases to activate a response of relaxation. As one engages in carrying out the specific body postures and poses while breathing deeply, the body then begins to shift from a state of tension and biochemical arousal to that of calm and relaxation. Deep breathing as you engage in a yoga pose helps in enhancing the response of the brain to threat. The body then begins to turn off nerve chemicals that trigger such response. For example the adrenaline then stops the dumping of sugar and fatty acids to the blood stream as a source of energy for the brain, muscles and the motor energy.

Realization of biochemical relaxation state helps with oxygenating the blood which then regulates overall health of the heart by bringing blood pressure, heart rate and motor activity to normal state. The yoga postures impacts all the body systems and apart from strengthening the muscles, it also tones the internal organs and the spine nerves. The practice of yoga also enhances the sense of self awareness as a person begins to cultivate a non judgmental relationship with one self. A person gets to exercise more and eat much healthier foods as the mind is active to alert them whenever they go wrong.

Below are of the benefits that are associated with practicing yoga;

## Physical Benefits

- Increased flexibility of the body

- Increased muscle tone and strength

- Improved energy, respiration and vitality

- Maintenance of balanced metabolism

- Loss of weight

- Cardiovascular and circulatory health.

- Improved athletic performance

- Protection from injury.

## Mental Benefits

- Improves behavior, moods and mindfulness.

- Improves wellbeing and resilience

- Increases body awareness and relieves stress.

- Reduces muscle tension, inflammation and strain.

- Enhances levels of concentration and attention

- Calms the body and centers the nervous system.

- Reduced impact of traumatic experience.

## Improvement of Flexibility

In the initial stages of yoga you will find that you are not able to touch certain parts of the body comfortably, as you go back to each and every time you soon realize that you will and it's a normal thing. The initial pains will also subside with time and the body then becomes much more flexible. The once un-coordinating parts of the body begin to coordinate for the better.

## Posture improvement

Poor posture is known to cause back pain and neck pains and can also contribute to muscle aches all over the body. On extreme cases they may cause arthritis of the spine and it's important to ensure that you do not confuse effects of poor posture with fatigue. Therefore as one become diligent in yoga it will ultimately result into posture improvement.

## Improved Muscle Strength

Stronger muscles are known to help is minimizing the risk of arthritis and back pains. Flabby muscles usually put pressure on the bones which may result into other complications. The good thing is that as you strengthen your muscles through practicing yoga which then leads to enhanced flexibility.

## Protection of the spine

Spinal disks are the points of movement to the spine and any discomfort to them can be so painful; therefore well coordinated backbends, forward bends and moderate twists will make the disks in good form.

## Enhanced Bone health

Yoga practice is an effective way to prevent osteoporosis which is brittle bones. Most of the yoga moves makes one to carry his own weight and therefore strengthening the bones. This also helps in keeping calcium in the bones.

## Increased blood flow

There is improved blood circulation with yoga because of the exercises involved. Increased blood flow, also result in increased oxygen flow in the body; yoga helps even to push deeper into the body oxygenated blood because some of these exercises like twisting penetrates better. It's been proven that inverted positions help the blood from the legs to flow back to the heart easily thereby making it easy to receive oxygen to be pumped to the rest of the body. Research has proved that yoga boosts levels of hemoglobin and red blood cells. It also thins blood and by that makes the blood platelets less sticky which in turn reduces the blood clot enhancing proteins. This is also a solution to issues of heart attack which are commonly due to blood clots.

## Prevention of Cartilage and weakening of Joints

Joints will always get to do full motions while on yoga, which in turn prevents arthritis. Joint cartilages receive nutrients when the fluid in them are squeezed out and replenished with new ones. When this process is not sustained then the joints risk wearing out and may expose the other bones.

## Better sleep

With a good yoga exercise you will realize that the body is more relaxed and the soul is at peace which is a good recipe for deep sleep. When the senses are turned inwards, even the nervous system will cool down thereby the body being able to get the much desired rest.

## Strong Immune system

The immune system in this case is not really due to the movements but it's derived from the meditation itself. It is meditation that drives deep and connects with the immune system and regulating it accordingly.

## Increases lung efficiency

When breathing is done through the nose as with yoga, the air gets filtered from dirt and other stuff that are carried in the air. It also aids in deep breathing which stretches the lungs to capacity and improves efficient exhalation.

## Improved digestion

Lack of enough body exercise at times may lead to constipation and other bowel challenges. Some of these also come as a result of stress and therefore by engaging in yoga practice all that stress is released. At the same time there is faster transportation of foods and waste through the canals.

## Positive self esteem

Self esteem is built and certain factors can contribute to low self esteem. At times poor physique can lead to it which in essence may lead to poor mental and spiritual health.

## Pain reliever

There are several pains that can be reduced by yoga, like arthritis, upper thoracic pains, fibromyalgia and some other chronic ailments. With less or no pains in the body, you have all the advantage of being active and involved with life.

## Inner Strength

When you seem like you are at a standstill then it becomes easy to realize change after a few sessions of yoga. You can literally feel life and a lot of inner strength; you will also realize that you are optimistic of possible outcomes to what you are pursuing in life. If well utilized it can help you get rid of the dysfunctional habits.

## Reduction of drugs

Given that yoga helps tackle milliards of problems in the human body, as you continue with it, it's possible that you can end up doing away with drugs and save money if you were dealing with a chronic disease.

## Transformation Awareness

Transformation is a function of the mind and given that yoga deals with the mind then as one gets deeper then he will be able to receive uncommon ideas on how to move forward. A transformed mind is able to process things differently. Yoga reduces anger when feelings of anger are suppressed and feelings of compassion are enhanced which then soothes the nervous system and the mind. With a strong mind it's easy to go through adversity and come out of it easily without being shaken by the adversity.

## Enhancing relationships

The principle of yoga borders on friendliness, equality and compassion amongst other things. Talking the truth and when given opportunity, you only take what you need, enhances friendships and relationships which makes people comfortable around you.

## Easy guidance

When practicing under a good guide, it becomes easier to ascend to better and higher levels as is desired by your tutor especially after being convinced that you are worth getting to the next level.

# Chapter 4

## Yoga Practice with examples and Pictures

As you begin yoga exercises its important to note that yoga practice entails less of exercises and more of mind and body exploration. Exercises therefore entail sweating as you also push the body into being in the exercise mode. The below exercises can be carried out in a meditative mode as they can have diverse impact to the body that may lead to success in the process.

### 1. Easy Pose

This is one of the comfortable seated position that's quite ideal for meditation purposes. This pose helps with opening of the hips while also lengthening the spine. The pose also enhances inner calm and grounding. In this exercise you are expected to sit with your legs crossed just as you did when you were a kid. All you have to do is to press your hips o the floor as you focus on the crown of your head for a lengthened spine. Let your shoulders drop back as you press your chest forward. Let your face, belly and jaws relax then breathe deeply through your nose all the way to your belly and as long as you may find it comfortable.

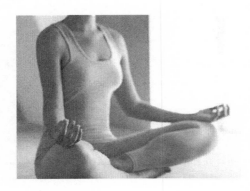

## 2. Downward Facing Dog

Once you're practiced the easy pose, you can progress to the downward facing dog as its one of the common and mostly recognized yoga poses. The exercise has that rejuvenating stretch that's quite essential for enhanced flexibility. Some of the benefits of the downward facing dog pose include;

- Helps with calming of the brain while also relieving stress and any mild depression.

- It energizes the body

- It stretches the shoulders, calves, hamstrings, hand and arches.

- Strengthens both arms and legs.

- Relieves from the symptoms of menopause

- Relieves from pains that are associated with menstrual discomfort.

- Prevents osteoporosis

- Improves digestion

- Relieves form back pain, fatigue, insomnia and headache.

- The exercise is therapeutic for asthmatic conditions, high blood pressure, sciatica and flat feet amongst others.

To practice the exercise place your hands and toes on the floor then exhale as you raise your knees from the floor. Walk your hands forward as you press your fingers wide with your palms pressing on the mat. Press your hips towards the ceiling as you as you bring your body into a V shape. You should also press your shoulders away from the ears. The knees should be slightly bent with. You can practice the exercise as you hold 3 full breaths.

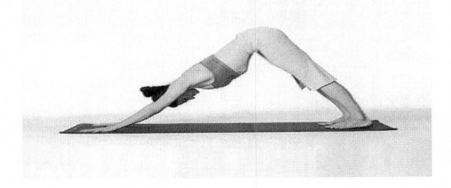

### 3. Sun salutations

Engaging in a few rounds of sun salutation exercise can have a great impact especially when you may not be having sufficient time to attend yoga classes. Below are the illustrations on how to go through the exercise.

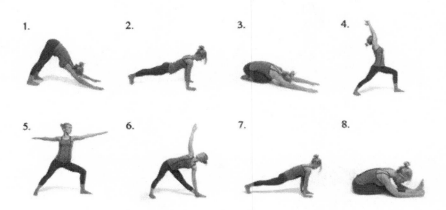

## 4. Tree Pose

To engage in this exercise stand with your arms at the sides then shift weight onto your left leg s you also place the sole of your right foot on the left thigh with the hips facing forward. Once your body is balanced, bring your hand as in a prayer position with palms together. As you breathe in, extend your arms above your shoulders with the palms facing each other for about 30 seconds. You can then lower your arms and repeat on the other side.

The benefits of tree pose include;

- Strengthening of the calves, ankles, thighs and the spine.

- It stretches the inner thighs and the groins, shoulders and the chest.

- It improves the sense of balance.

- Reduces flat feet while also relieving sciatica.

The aim of this exercise is to be able to achieve the firmness and rootedness of a tree and engaging in regular practice has a way of enhancing balance and coordination while also improving concentration.

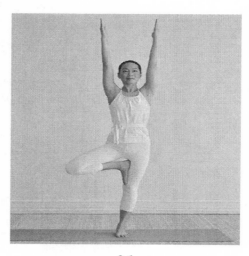

## 5. Extended Triangle Pose

This exercise can be practiced by extending the arms out to the sides as you bend over your right leg. You can then stand with your feet apart and the toes on your right foot twisted to 90 degrees and the left foot at 45 degree. Let your right hand touch the floor as you rest on the right leg or above the knee. You can also extend your left hand fingertips toward the ceiling. Gaze towards the ceiling as you hold 5 breaths. Stand and then repeat on the opposite side.

Benefits of triangle pose are:

- Strengthens and stretches the thighs ankles and knees.

- Stretches the hips hamstrings, groins, shoulders, calves, chest and spine.

- Stimulates abdominal organs.

- Relieves stress

- Relieves menopause symptoms

- Relieves backache, therapeutic for anxiety, neck pain and more.

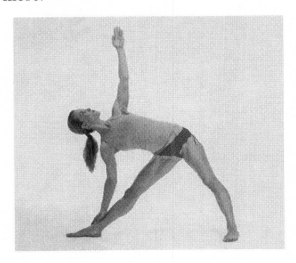

## 6. Seated forward bend

To practice the pose sit on the floor with your legs straight in front then press through your heels as you turn your thighs slightly in as shown in the picture below.

The benefits of seated forward bend are:

- Calms the brain while also relieving mild depression and tress.

- Stretches the spine, hamstrings and shoulders

- Stimulates the kidneys, liver, uterus and ovaries.

- Improves digestion amongst others.

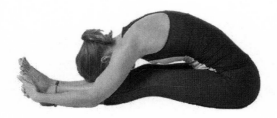

## 7. Wide angle seated forward bend

Start the exercise by stretching your legs to 90 degrees as you sit straight. You can alternate by leaning forwards and backwards as you control your breathing just as demonstrated below.

The benefits of the exercise are;

- Stretches both the insides and back of the legs.

- Stimulates abdominal organs

- Strengthens the spine

- Calms the brain

- Releases groins.

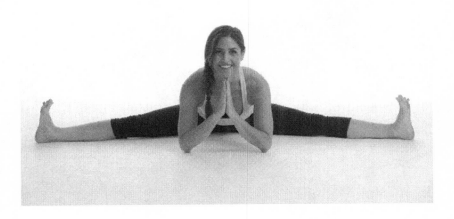

## 8. Full boat pose

Sit on the floor with your legs straight and turn the thighs to 45 degrees as you inhale and exhale. Your hands should stretch straight above your thighs as demonstrated below. The benefits of full boat pose are;

- Strengthens the abdomen, spine and hip flexors

- Stimulates the kidneys prostrate glands, intestines and thyroid.

- Helps relieve stress

- Improves digestion

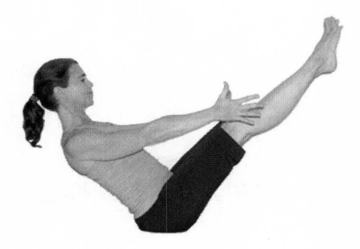

## 9. Bridge Pose

To practice this exercise, clasp your hands under the lower back as you press your arms down. Lift your hips until the thighs as you bring your chest towards the chin. Hold on it for a minute as you exhale. Benefits of this pose are;

- It rejuvenates tired legs.

- Stretches the things while also extending the spine amongst other benefits.

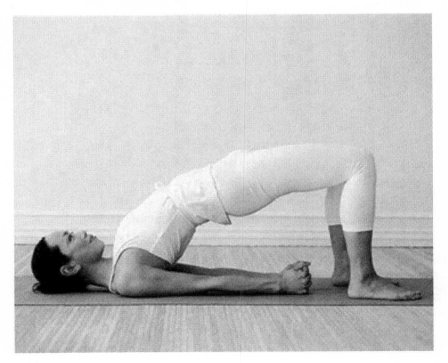

# How often does one need to practice Yoga

When it comes to practicing yoga and realizing your desired goals and expected benefits, it's important to note that there is no quick fix to yoga. If you are to realize the desired results then you have to commit the time and discipline to practice. Yoga is known as an al encompassing practice that creates a connection between the mind and the body. Achievement of the desired results takes commitment and dedication and that can be frustrating to a person that's used to getting quick fixes.

Commitment to a regular practice routine is therefore very vital if you are to realize tangible improvements in terms of coordination, strength and flexibility, and balance amongst others. Consistent practice is what enhances body awareness as you intelligently progress with the process. If you dedicate your practice to only one a week then sustaining that level of awareness can be a challenge. It may also feel like you're starting afresh whenever you begin the practice. Realizing tangible progress with once a week routine for practice may not bring the desired results.

If you have a challenge then you can schedule so that your practice time takes shorter time like between 15-30 minutes. It's when you commit to a daily practice even if it's for 15 minutes that you will be able to realize results. If you can get time daily to practice then you will be able to realize your desired results much faster than a person who only practices once a week.

# Chapter 5

## Practicing Meditation

Meditation is a form of relaxation that's practiced with the aim of reaching a state of serenity within the body and the mind. It's usually an easy process but may not be that obvious for beginners. Some of the things to work on are breathing and learning to remove things that clutter the mind. You need to have a lot of practice to know how to clear the mind. When one is able to attain this then it then becomes easy to reach peace, calmness, and serenity thereby opening you to fresh insights. It's necessary to know that you do not have right and wrong when undertaking meditation. The thing is that all answers are within us that are able to address all universal concerns. There is no particular age that should get engaged in meditation but the whole thing can be guided by parents in cases involving children.

It's been said that it's not possible to teach someone how to meditate just as it's not easy to teach someone how to fall asleep. Just like sleep which catches us whenever we stay detached to various mental concerns, meditation equally cannot be forced. It's a conscious state that can be attained through observing heightened awareness and strong will power. To achieve that meditative state it's important that one gets to relax by letting go of all forms of anxieties and desires. The subtle balance that's required between detachment from all manner of distractions and effort necessary to maintain concentration is what can be described as the art of meditation.

To attain that meditative state it's important that one gets to learn how to have the mind focused without having any struggle. One should get prepared and there are various steps that should be taken into consideration if the process of meditation is to be realized. Below are some of the steps that can be followed for an effective process of meditation;

## 1. The Place

The place where you choose to practice meditation can have a great impact on how the process turns out. It's important that you have a specific place where you can carry out meditation like a special room. If it's not possible to have a whole room dedicated for meditation then you can apportion a space within the room. The place should be kept clean and tidy and should be maintained as a place that's only used for meditation. The place should be free from any form of distractions and only those who value its sacredness should be allowed to access the place.

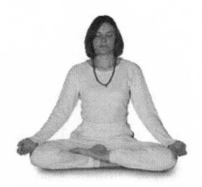

## 2. The Place of Focus

Set up a place of focal point within the room that you can focus on. For example, you can place a table in the room with an oil lamp or a candle. Light is a spiritual symbol and gazing at a flame while starting off meditation helps with enhancing the process. Gazing at the light steadily is equally an exercise on its own. You can also place a flower vase with flowers o the table as it creates feelings of joy in the mind. There are those who incorporate the process of meditation with burning incense as a way of purifying the room and enhancing the energy within the space. The practice however depends on one's spiritual persuasion and belief. In case you prefer burning incense then opt for natural incense such as use of sandalwood given its cooling and calming effect that it has on the mind. A religious person can place a spiritual symbol that's aligned to your spiritual belief.

You can also choose a place like meditating in nature while facing the ocean, river, mountain, under the tree or while facing the rising or setting of the sun.

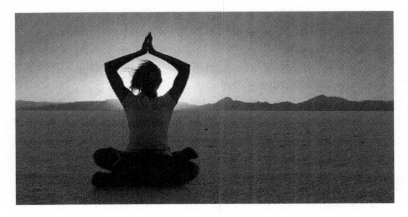

### 3. The Time

The best time for engaging in meditation is either at dawn or dusk as that's the time when the atmosphere is mostly charged with spiritual force. Right after sleep you will find that the mind is quiet with the atmosphere very clear without interference from the day activities. Concentration at this time becomes easy and effortless and if this time is not appropriate for you then you can choose times that that you find appropriate for you. Evening time is also appropriate especially before going to bed. You need a time when the mind is freed from most of the tensions that one gets to accumulate all through the day.

### 4. The Habit of Meditation

Without developing a habit of consistent meditation, you may not be able to realize the benefits that come with the practice. Maintaining consistency alongside meditating everyday at the same time is important if you want to develop the habit of meditating. It's much better to meditate every day for about 30 minutes than dedicating more time to meditate once in a week. Once you develop the habit, you will realize that you experience some level of discomfort whenever you fail to just as it is whenever on fails to take bath. Meditation can be compared to medical cleansing that' suitable for the overall mental well being of an individual. Once you begin to experience discomfort whenever you miss practice, you will then become more committed to the practice.

### 5. The sitting position

To start the process well, you need to sit in a comfortable position with a steady posture. Your neck and spine should be erect and not tensed. Your psychic current should be able to freely travel from the base of your spine to the top of your head for enhanced concentration and steady mind. Sitting in a crossed legged position helps with providing the body with a firm base however you may wish to sit in a position that you find to be appropriate and comfortable.

Remember to sit in a position that allows for the effective flow of energy and a triangular position is ideal as it enables the energy to disperse to various directions within the body. Try sitting in a way that enables the body to relax especially the face, neck and shoulder muscles.

As you practice yoga postures consistently, you will be able to keep the back straight and be comfortable with any position that you may want to try. Practicing yoga helps with eliminating the feelings of fatigue as the meditation state is expected to be firm and pleasant. The practices make your body to be at ease without requiring any attention during the meditation process. Once the body is at ease, one is able to disconnect from the awareness of being the body and will get to easily focus on deeper aspects self consciousness. Remember that you may not be perfect from a few trials but mastery will be attained as you continue to remain consistent with the practice. Achieving the right meditative posture will give you confidence in regards to overcoming greater obstacles.

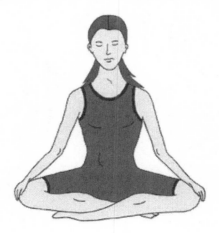

# The Breath

Practice the process of relaxing and allowing rhythmic breathing. You can begin with a minute of deep abdominal breath that has the potential of bringing sufficient oxygen to the brain. You can also practice slowing your breath down as you inhale and exhale rhythmically. This technique according to yoga practice is called pranayama which refers to breath control and the exercises are aimed at steadying the breath which then calms the mind. Meditation enables us to see things as clear as they are without the influence of our perceptions of likes and dislikes. Detachment from any forms of hope and fear protects against any form of suffering which then acts as a way of making a commitment to your well being.

By gently disciplining your mind to be quiet for a given period of time as you focus on the present moment you will realize that your life gets immeasurably enhanced.

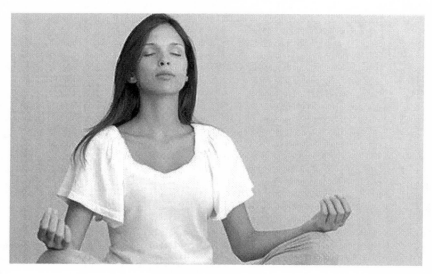

# The Mind

For the practice of meditation to be effective you will need to transform your mind by eliminating any form of negativity and suffering as you welcome broad vision, joy, heightened awareness and a sense of contentment into your life. The extent of your success will be commensurate to how you are committed to the goal. For real change to take place you will need to understand that commitment to a goal does not in any way limit freedom. Try to confine the mind to only focus on the desired energy centre as meditation is more of a heart commitment and where your heart goes the mind gets to follow.

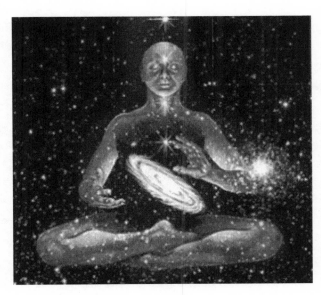

# Choose a point of Concentration

As you engage in meditation, choose a given focal point where the mind can rest. The mind requires an anchorage point where it can be grounded given a lot of time is spent on daydreaming and being disconnected from the moment. This can be achieved by having awareness to the body posture and breath. It can also be strengthened by focusing attention to a particular point within the body and these points are referred to as chakras or the body energy centers. There is a branch of raja yoga which focuses on the energy centers and how the energies can be released for the expansion of consciousness.

There are seven main energy centers in the body and other secondary ones. The energy centers correspond to levels of consciousness differently with the three lower energy centers responding mostly to desires of the mind that are basic like that for security, pleasure and expression of individuality. The forth which is the heart energy center corresponds to expression of love; the throat energy center is where the consciousness expands to incorporate knowledge of both the past and future lives.

The sixth one is located between the eyebrows and is known as the place for institutional knowledge. The last energy centre which is on top of the head I responsible for a state of union with the comic consciousness. For meditation purposes, it's recommended that one gets to focus on the heart centre which according to yoga practice is the anahata chakra. People with emotional kind of personality are also encouraged to focus on the heart energy center as it may make it easier for towards channeling more emotional energy which then leads to manifestation of selfless love.

If you have a personality that's predominantly intellectual then it's vital that you focus at the energy center between the eyebrows which is the center responsible for self awareness. Focusing more on the energy center will release will gradually release it from having a narrow and selfish vision. Your intuition will open up and you may be able to perceive reality clearly without the influence of any limitation caused by the intellect. The state is also referred to as the opening of the third eye. The main point here is to be able to train your energies in order to stabilize at one point. It's important to keep the energy at the same place as changing it may lead to instability which leads to the wandering of the mind. The energy should be trained to flow in a specific way. Focusing your mind is what leads to concentration which then allows the mind to focus more into the infinite space.

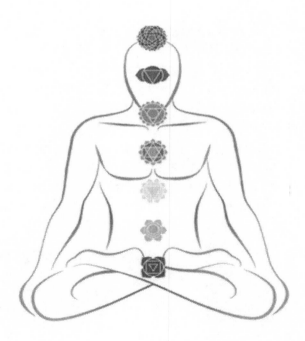

# Choosing an object to concentrate on

Even as you get into deep meditation you will need to continue with stabilization of your mental energy. The mind therefore require training on concentration and for that to be achieved an object of focus should be used. Concentration is attained when one has a firm posture with a slow breath and focus on a given energy centre. However this is still just a process of meditation and not the actual meditation. Being in a state f meditation is when the mind is beyond that state of concentration and that can only be realized through a concentrated mind. There are yoga practices that recommend use of mantras or words that have power as a tool to enhance concentration. The mantra can be repeated mentally while also synchronizing with the breath and all should be harnessed to become one point.

Mantra helps with focusing the desire to see and to hear, aspects of the mind that have the potential of interrupting the flow of energy if not well harmonized. As you repeat the sound you get to visualize it even as you listen to it. You can then focus on any symbol that you may prefer as per your religious beliefs or any other thing that you may be comfortable focusing on. The object of your focus should be something that's uplifting and with the ability of enabling your mind shift to the infinite. Things like the sun, light or the sky can be considered of religious symbols like of Buddha, the cross or OM can also be focused on.

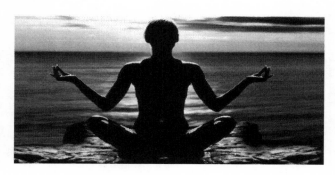

# Giving Space to the Mind

As you engage in concentration try not to force your mind as it will start by wondering but will then settle into concentration. If you focus too hard on getting your mind to concentrate then you may develop some mild headache which is not appropriate. What you need to do is to relax deeply as you focus on your breath. Try to avoid the desire of having a quick fix and instead remember that there isn't an easy way of bringing your mind to focus and concentration. The mind should gradually be freed from the numerous layers of emotional burden.

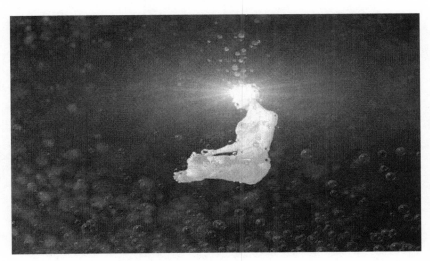

# Disassociating from the Mind

If the mind persistently continue with wondering then what you can do is to disassociate from it and watch it from distance. The mind can at times be resistant and may continue to wonder in the world of imagination, a fact that can be quite frustrating. Disassociating from the mind can therefore be of great help in helping the mind to gradually slow down as you also try to stop feeding the emotions and thoughts through your consciousness. Emotional strength is required if the separation is to be maintained. As much as the practice may prove to be a bit demanding for a beginner by engaging in practice consistently, one is able to realize success with the practice of meditation.

Pure thought is attained as a result of sustained concentration which then leads to meditation. This state may be achieved after engaging in practice for months. Remember it's by sustained meditation that one gets to enter into a state where the mind finds absorption in consciousness. This is the highest state of consciousness where duality disappears and one gets to enter a state of super consciousness.

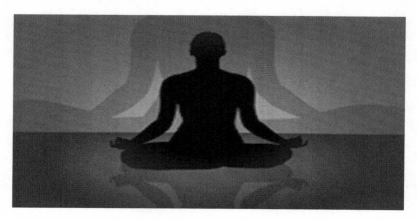

# Types of Meditation
## 1. Universal Mantra Meditation

This type of meditation as we shared earlier can be quite easy yet very powerful when well practiced. This is where a mantra is used as an object of focus ad a mantra can be a phrase or a word that has the potential of shifting deeper into more peaceful levels of awareness. The mantra should be repeated faintly and gently in the mind. This technique becomes powerful when you let go of any other thought as you allow your attention to get into deeper levels of awareness.

To practice this you should follow the steps below:

- Sit down comfortably with your spine straight and eyes closed. Begin to repeat the mantra in your mind gently. It can be an affirmation like "My life is getting better day by day" or words like "Aum" or any phrase that you desire.

- Let the mantra arise faintly through your mind as you begin to repeat it with less effort. Continue with the repletion until you begin to feel like you're slipping into a state of sleep then allow that to happen.

- Once you realize that your attention has drifted from the mantra begin to repeat it again for about 10 minutes then slowly begin to come out of the meditation.

## 2. Relaxation Meditation

This method of meditation is quite easy and it involves use of the eyes. To practice this meditation you can engage in the following;

- Sit in a comfortable place with your spine straight. Let your eyes to comfortably res downward as you softly gaze without focusing on anything.

- Let your eyelids drop to a comfortable level without closing your eyes as you continue to gaze downwards. Your primary focus should be gazing and you will realize that your breathing becomes more rhythmic.

- If your eyes get very heavy hen you can let them close and if you realize that your attention has drifted then get back to that downward gaze.

### 3. Energy healing meditation

This form of meditation entails sending the powerful healing force to the area that you want help in. The life force is the energy is the energy that flows behind all the healing and whenever it flows there will be balance, well being and health. The goal here is to concentrate your positive energy on the area that's afflicted and to practice this;

- Sit straight and close your eyes, as you breathe silently and slowly.

- As you inhale feel like you're breathing in the healing force right through your solar plexus as you picture it as a refined light energy.

- As you exhale, direct this light gently to the afflicted area and if there isn't any afflicted area then disperse the light all through your body.

- Continue with the process until you feel that the intended area has received sufficient life force.

### 4. Color healing meditation

We are not just physical beings but multidimensional beings and this meditation is intended to harmonize all our bodies the spiritual, mental, physical and emotional bodies. Color healing meditation provides the cleansing, healing and balancing at all levels of the body.

To practice the process;

- Sit comfortably with closed eyes as you visualize a ball of golden light over your head. Visualize the ball of light descend through the crown of your head as it fills the entire body with the golden light.

- Imagine yourself absorbing the light as it nourishes, heals and cleanses your entire being. Your spirit and body should be able to dissolve the blocked toxic energies.

- Repeat the exercise with different types of light and then take time to visualize yourself in a perfect state and with radiant health.

## 5. Centering

Centering can be defined as meditation in action. Within every person is that place that's always peaceful and calm and to be centered means you remain in that cal centre regardless of the things around your life. To be centered means you don't allow that inner light to get overshadowed with negative thoughts and stressful circumstances. While in that state you get to experience, focus, peace, clarity, balance and such like. When you're not centered you're likely to experience lack of clarity, stress, lack of focus and such like.

Below are some of the centering techniques:
- Simple breath awareness
- Reclaiming your energy
- Letting go
- Allow the inflow of subtle energy

# Conclusion

Congratulations and thank you for taking your time to read the book all through. I know you've gathered valuable information from the book and that may not have any impact unless you go ahead and implement what you have read. Remember that a lot of information has been shared in this book and implementing it in its entirety can be overwhelming.

It's advisable that you only implement it bit by bit. You can pick one exercise or two and work on them until you feel that you're efficient in them. As for the meditation exercises, you can pick on each at a time then try out and if you find that which works well for you then you can stay with it.

Thank you so much for taking your time to read the book all through and I have a small request, kindly go ahead and live a good review for the book.

Thank you

Made in the USA
Middletown, DE
02 January 2018